VERRUCAE

CAUSE AND TREATMENT

BY THE SAME AUTHOR

The Pathomechanics of Abnormal Pronation

Published by Open Study Group Ltd

VERRUCAE

CAUSE AND TREATMENT

The history, diagnosis and treatment of verrucae
from 1907 to the present day

by

E E H Wietscher

FSSCh

Open Study Group

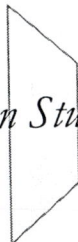

Acknowledgements

My grateful thanks go to Peter J Read and Franklin Charlesworth respectively, for the vast amount of information contained in their books *Therapeutics for Chiropodists* and *Chiropody Theory and Practice*, so essential to my research. I believe the former book is still available but the latter out of print. Both books have rightly been considered 'required reading' over the years: I cannot argue with that verdict.

CONTENTS

1907 to the 1940s 9
  Aetiology 9
  The Virus Theory 9
  The Traumatic Theory 10
  The Psychological Factor 10
  Hypnotic Suggestion 11
  The Current View 12
  Differential Diagnosis 12

Defence Mechanisms of the Body 15
  Basic Types of Wound Repair 17
  How Blood Helps in the Healing Process 18
  Cell Mediated Immunity (CMI) 19

Types of Wart 21
  Long Standing Plantar Warts (a note of warning) 23

Treatment of Warts (Verrucae) 25

Types of Treatment 26
  Drugs 26
  X-ray Therapy 26
  Electro-surgery and Fulguration 27
  Cryosurgery 28
  Chemical Cautery 29
  Use of Drugs in Chemical Cautery 30
  For the Treatment of Callus 31

Glossary of Common Terms 45

Photographic Plates 51

1907 to the 1940s

Verruca, or plantar wart, is a benign growth highly vascular in nature, which involves not only the epidermis but also the derma.

Verrucae can be found on any part of the body but most common situations are on hands and feet. Those which occur on the feet can generally be divided into two types: verruca arida (dry type) and verruca humida (moist type).

Aetiology

The aetiology of warts still fuels much discussion. Many in the medical profession take the attitude 'leave them alone and they will go away by themselves'. This has caused many problems for chiropodists who generally feel that treating them is by far the best way to deal with them.

To understand more fully the need for treatment or indeed the need not to treat them, we need to look closely at what is known of the genesis of verrucae and their treatment.

The Virus Theory

Variot first demonstrated the infective nature of these growths in 1893; he showed that warts were auto-inoculable and transmissible.

In 1907 Cuiffe showed that the infective agent could be passed through a bacterial filter.

Wile and Kingery in 1921 further supported the theories of Variot and Cuiffe by producing verrucae experimentally from a filter passing virus. The verrucae were crushed and put into a solution, which was then filtered through a very fine filter (too fine to allow passage of bacterium). The subsequent filtrate proved to be capable of giving rise to growth of a verruca in living tissue.

The long incubation period after experimental inoculation led researchers to support the theory of virus infection. This factor was commented on by Templeton in 1935.

The prolonged incubation period of virus diseases is well known and is considerably in excess of most bacterial infections. In some instances the incubation period of experimentally produced warts extended up to twenty months.

An interesting factor brought to our attention by Roxburgh in *Common Skin Diseases,* seventh edition 1944, is the suggestion that all types of warts arise from the same virus. He states: "It also appears that all the varieties of wart mentioned are due to the same virus for inoculation of a filtrate of common warts may produce plane warts or common warts, and a filtrate of condylomata acuminate may produce common warts."

The Traumatic Theory

The Traumatic Theory is expounded for us by Franklin Charlesworth in his book *Chiropody Theory and Practice.* Under the heading 'Skin Diseases VERRUCAE' he has this to say: 'The traumatic origin of warts would appear to be amply illustrated by the numerous cases coming before the chiropodist. With only a few exceptions the primary growth occurs over pressure areas." The author propounds the theory that "both the infective and the traumatic origin of growths are tenable. It is that the local stimulus induces an excessive proliferation of prickle cell layer with an arresting of the normal process of cell degeneration. This may well be either of traumatic or infective origin. Both types of lesion have one factor in common, namely, an acute irritation of the prickle cell layer inducing mitosis."

The Psychological Factor

It is realised that in considering this feature we are moving away from the solid scientific ground of the virus and the traumatic theories into what may be called the mystic. Nevertheless, today there are many learned authorities that are not prepared to dismiss this type of approach:

"Ashen tree, ashen tree, pray you buy these warts from me"

to be repeated twice followed by the sticking of a pin into the tree which was then withdrawn and stuck into the wart. The pin was then removed from the wart and stuck back into the tree where it remained presumably until it dropped off the tree, which we presume is when the wart fell off the foot.

There are of course, many other methods, one of which was to rub the wart with a piece of steak first six times counter clockwise and then six times clockwise. The steak was then buried in the garden. As the steak rotted away so did the wart.

There are still people in country districts who claim to be able to buy warts from you, or just simply wish them away.

Hypnotic Suggestion

Hypnotic suggestion is another means put forward to help in the removal of warts.

In his 'Notes of a Biology Watcher' Lewis Thomas in *The Medusa and The Snail* notes that warts can be hypnotised away. He quotes controlled experiments of warts being cured by use of hypnosis. "A group of sufferers were hypnotised and instructed to cure the warts on one side of the body only: this duly happened." Lewis here strikes a delightfully human note when he states: "It is interesting that most warts vanished precisely as instructed, but it is even more fascinating that mistakes were made. Just as you might expect in other affairs requiring a clear understanding of which is left and which right, one of the subjects got mixed up and destroyed the warts on the wrong side."

Quite a thought-provoking idea. Imagine, if we had a clear understanding of how this worked, we would understand the identity of the cellular and chemical participants in tissue rejection, conceivably with some added information about the ways in which viruses create foreignness in cells.

We would have come to understand how the traffic of these reactants is directed, and then perhaps be able to understand the nature of certain diseases in which the traffic is being conducted in the wrong direction, so causing tissue destruction aimed at the wrong cells.

What can be learned from the above is that to be successful in treating verrucae, a Positive Mental Attitude (PMA) has to be developed not only by the patient but also by the practitioner.

Charlesworth states: "Many orthodox doctors now state that the success of many forms of treatment depends solely on the practitioner's faith in the treatment." In any case it does none of us any harm to give it the benefit of the doubt, and adopt a fully positive approach to our treatment regime.

The Current View

Verrucae are currently defined as common, contagious, epithelial tumours caused by the human papillomavirus (HPV) (derived from the Latin *papilla,* 'nipple', and the Greek suffix *-oma*). The human papilloma virus group (HPVG) has a large number of subtypes, at least a hundred, producing a large number of clinical pathologies, some of which can become malignant. *(Viral Infections of the Skin, The Merck Manual.)* Viral warts may appear at any age, but are most frequent in older children and uncommon although not unheard of in elderly people.

Appearance and size depend on their location and on the degree of irritation and trauma to which they are subjected. The course may be erratic. Infection may persist as single or multiple lesions, and lesions may develop by auto-inoculation.

Complete regression after several months is usual with or without treatment, but warts may persist for years and may reoccur at the same or at different sites.

Differential Diagnosis

The wart viruses are circular, double stranded DNA, with about 8000 base pairs. To qualify as a separate type there must be <50% of DNA cross-hybridization; for sub-types, >50%.

Each type is indicated by a number and, in general, causes certain clinical lesions. Although each DNA is distinctive, most papillomas, including those of bovine origin, also have a common protein antigen that can be demonstrated histologically on fixed tissue with a test that is positive for all types of papillomas and is very useful in diagnosis.

When papillomas become malignant, however, they no longer give a positive stain nor can recognisable particles be seen with the electron microscope.

Oncogenic papilloma DNA can then be found in cancers by modern molecular hybridization DNA techniques. DNA typing has become much more available in recent years and is important for prognosis of genital warts and their consequences.

Defence Mechanisms of the Body

One of the obvious basic features of man's existence is the fact that his external environment is often hostile and unfavourable from the moment of birth and abounds with potentially dangerous micro-organisms: bacteria, viruses, and other unicellular and multicellular parasites. These micro-organisms: (1) cause cellular damage directly by releasing enzymes that break down cell membranes and organelles; (2) give off toxins that act throughout the body to disrupt organs and tissues as well as the neuromuscular system; and (3) continue a steady drain of the body's energy supplies since some (viruses in particular) often take hold of the metabolic and reproductive mechanisms of the cell they inhabit.

The body's first line of defence against infection is the anatomic barrier of the surface exposed to the environment, that is the skin and mucous membranes.

The skin covering the weight-bearing plantar area of the foot is very much thicker than skin to be found elsewhere on the body or even on other non-weight bearing areas of the foot. The plantar stratum corneum (SC) is over 60 times thicker than that to be found on the abdomen. This is a result of larger numbers of cells being present; also these stratum corneum cells can in themselves be up to 30 times thicker than the less keratinised non-weight bearing SC cells to be found in other sites. This in part accounts for lesions, which are very distinct from lesions produced by the same pathogen on other skin sites.

Few micro-organisms can penetrate intact skin. Furthermore, sebaceous and sweat glands secrete chemicals that are toxic to certain bacteria, and mucous membranes contain antimicrobial chemicals as well as having sticky mucus where ciliary action sweeps the organism away or where phagocytic cells can engulf them. Thus, our major defence is the 'unbroken' cover or shield of skin and mucous membranes. If the skin is penetrated or burned, there is a serious loss of body fluids and the body works rapidly to close openings. The blood provides its own plug or clot as we shall see later, and the surrounding tissues repair themselves. However, in spite of the body's external defence surfaces, small pathogenic (disease-producing) micro-organisms do enter. They cause illness either by disrupting body cells or by producing toxins (poisons).Their effects are often specific and affect a limited area in a certain way. For example, the bacteria causing diphtheria produce toxin that acts on the heart muscle and some motor neurons; therefore, they must be completely destroyed or their toxins neutralised. Several defence mechanisms are in operation, the most important being the chemical substances referred to as antibodies, and these complement a group of specialised phagocytic cells. One of the body's unique aspects is its ability to recognise and destroy any substance recognised as foreign protein.

Due to the fact that the majority of treatment regimes for HPV will induce destruction of tissue it is important at this time to gain a little understanding of how the body repairs itself. We will start with the skin. How is it made up?

Epidermis (epi 'on', derma 'skin')

The outer epithelial portion of the skin. The palms and soles have the following strata:

a) Stratum corneum (horny layer)
b) Stratum lucidum (clear layer) (in other parts of the body stratum lucidum may not be present)
c) Stratum granulosum (granular layer)
d) Stratum basale (basal layer)

Dermis or corium

Cutis vera; enderon; a layer of skin composed of a superficial thin layer that interdigitates with the epidermis, the stratum papillare, and the stratum reticulare. It contains blood and lymphatic vessels, nerves and nerve endings, glands, and except for glabrous skin, hair follicles.

What happens to the skin when it is cut?

Usually there is a vasoconstriction that occurs first. It is very transient, lasting only five or ten minutes. This is followed by the body's attempt to prevent hypovolemic shock. This is followed by an intense vasodilation where mast cells and histamine release cause the venules to expand releasing polymorphonuclearcytes (PPMs) and macrophages into the wound to set the stage for the removal of debris. This initial stage lasts approximately three to four days.

Basic Types of Wound Repair

There are three basic phases of wound repair:

a) Inflammatory 10%
b) Fibroblastic 20%
c) Maturation 70%

Inflammatory

The first is the inflammatory phase. It is also called the 'substrate' or 'lag' phase. The term 'lag' is a misnomer because a tremendous amount of activity is beginning at this time. Every wound needs inflammation to move the healing constituents into the area. Excessive inflammation produces swelling and pain.

Fibroblastic

The second phase of wound healing is called the 'fibroblastic' phase, migratory phase or proliferative phase. This phase lasts approximately three weeks. It begins roughly when the inflammatory phase stops. Tensile strength begins now with the synthesis of collagen. This synthesis is very active around the sixth day of healing and reaches 35% of its original strength at the fourteenth day. Since the tensile strength of the wound now equals the tensile strength of sutures, any sutures can be removed at this stage. This 35% is not an adequate strength if the skin margins were to be pulled apart at this time, so the use of steri-strips can help hold the edges together while the wound gains in strength. Studies have shown that a wound never reaches its original strength: 80% appears to be the maximum. It has also been proven that tension on a wound stimulates production of collagen, which initially is beneficial, but later in wound healing, lysis of collagen is needed to produce a pleasing scar.

By removing excessive tension with the use of a paper skin strip, we can help prevent the formation of a hypertrophic scar.

Maturation

The third phase of wound repair is called maturation. This phase begins after the fibroblastic phase ends and lasts up to a year. The changes in this phase take place slowly in comparison to those of the other two phases. Scar remodelling is taking place. After two months the scar may look thick but usually by six months it will look acceptable. Only after six months and preferably not before a year do we know what a scar will look like. If revision of a scar is contemplated, most surgeons suggest six months as the earliest time that this revision should take place and preferably not until after one year.

One final concept to remember is that these three phases are not cut and dried. They do not end and begin at precise moments but, in fact, overlap. By understanding this and the functions of each phase, we can assist wound healing as opposed to hindering it.

How Blood Helps in the Healing Process

When an injury occurs the body's first-aid mechanisms automatically begin to operate. The blood vessels in the neighbourhood of the injury dilate to provide an increased blood supply. At the same time the pores in the thin walls of the capillaries widen, letting more plasma than usual flow through to the injured tissues. The immediate result is twofold: the increased flow of blood and plasma brings the body's repair materials to the spot in large quantities and the increase in fluid at the spot distends tissues, presses on nerves and raises the local temperature. This whole process is called inflammation. It is one of the body's protective devices. Inflammation causes pain, which impairs the function of the injured part.

Blood clotting

If the skin is broken and there is bleeding, another mechanism, blood clotting, goes into operation at the site of the injury. Twelve essential clotting substances or factors are recognised. Of the four chief ones, only three are ordinarily present in the blood; the fourth is locked into the tissues. Not until tissue is damaged and the fourth substance is liberated is the blood clotting or coagulating mechanism put to work.

In the blood there are fragments of protoplasm known as platelets. Even though no more than a few drops of blood may flow from a cut, platelets by the tens of thousands come into contact with the rough edge of injured tissue and they disintegrate. Thus they liberate thromboplastin. This acts upon one of the constituents of the blood, prothrombin, and in the presence of calcium, also a normal constituent of the blood, the prothrombin changes to a similar but active material, thrombin. Now the newly formed thrombin reacts with another chemical in the blood, fibrinogen, to form fibrin. This substance, the end product of the series of chemical reactions, is insoluble and sponge–like and has the property of being able to contract. It forms a network of threads that enmesh the erythrocytes; it pulls them together as it contracts into a tough mass called a clot, which acts like a cork to stop up the opening. The platelets help to stop the flow of blood in two additional ways. They release a chemical that stimulates the muscle walls of nearby blood vessels to contract, narrowing the channels along which the blood flows to the cut and also narrowing the cut end that needs to be plugged. Also, the platelets themselves, being sticky, act as a natural adhesive, helping to seal up the cut. They are both chemical and mechanical agents.

The same materials that arrest bleeding prepare the site for mending. The fibrin threads contract and pull together the edges of the wound under the natural adhesive patch of the clot, and the repair cells go to work. These repair cells are a variety of connective tissue, long and spindle shaped with fibrous branches; they bind the edges of the wound neatly together. This done, their work is ended; their remnants and the remnants of cells damaged in the injury are cleared away by scavenger cells (phagocytes), cellular sanitation squads that keep all kinds of microscopic debris from cluttering the body tissues.

Cell Mediated Immunity (CMI)

When destruction of cells occurs as in chemical, drug or cryo-surgery regimes intended to treat HPV, cell particles are released into surrounding tissue. These may comprise virus particles, in this case HPV particles, and tissue particles present due to destruction of tissue: these are termed *antigens*. The body's response to these antigens is to produce antibodies, which will destroy the relevant rogue or foreign material. Along with macrophages other helper cells rush to clear the area. Among these are lymphocytes. While lymphocyte B cells are immunologically important they are not thymus dependant and are short lived. Responsible for the production of immunoglobulins, they are the precursor of the plasma cell and do not play a role in cell mediated immunity. T cells, however, are thermocyte-derived lymphocytes and are of immunological importance; they are long lived (months or years) and are responsible for cell mediated immunity.

Non-thymic lymphocytes, which kill virus-infected cells and cancer cells, do not need prior antigen activation in order to work and are therefore the body's first line of defence. Cytotoxic T cells, however, must first be activated by the presence of antigens. These sensitised T cells then undergo enlargement and multiplication over a 1-2 week period. This time lag is responsible for the delayed hypersensitivity reaction of CMI. When these cytotoxic T cells bind with the surface antigen of the infected cells this triggers the release of lymphokines resulting in target cell lysis. Cytotoxic T cells and NK cells (Langerhans cells) are recruited, activated and enhanced by intelukin-2 (IL2), a T cell growth factor from helper T cells. Interferon, produced by most body cells, is also brought into the picture at this time. All of these actions and reactions form part of the body's auto-immune system. The body will normally produce many more of these cells than are actually required. As many of these cells are of the long life variety they remain in the body ready to fight the next infection of this type that comes along.

We are all aware that some patients have an auto-immune system that does not work. These patients are susceptible to any infections either bacterial, fungal or viral.

Special drugs and treatments have been devised to help this type of patient. However as these types of drug and the treatments associated with them are not available to those working outside the confines of a hospital department, I will go no further on this subject, excepting of course, that there are patients whose immune response is completely normal to most bacteria, fungal and viral infections with the exception of certain ones as in EV infection usually caused by HPV8.

Types of Wart

The Common Wart (Verruca Vulgaris)

Common warts are almost universal in the population and most do not become malignant. They are sharply demarcated (the foot/hand print disappearing), rough surfaced, round or irregular, firm, light grey, yellow, brown, or greyish black tumours readily palpable, 2 to 10 mm in diameter. They appear most frequently on sites subject to trauma (eg fingers, elbows, knees, face, and scalp) but may be spread elsewhere. Periungal Warts are common warts occurring around the nail plate.

Filiform warts

Filiform warts are long, narrow, small growths usually seen on the eyelids, face, neck or lips.

Flat warts

Flat warts are smooth, flat, yellow-brown lesions and occur more commonly in children and young adults, most often on the face and along scratch marks through auto-inoculation.

Warts of unusual shape

Warts of unusual shape eg, pedunculated, or resembling a cauliflower, are most frequent on the head and neck, especially on the scalp and beard region although as shown in one of the accompanying photographs they can also be present on the foot.

Plantar warts

Plantar warts are common warts on the sole of the foot; they are flattened by pressure and surrounded by cornified epithelium. They may be exquisitely tender especially when squeezed between thumbs. They may be distinguished between corns and callous by their tendency to pinpoint bleeding when the surface is pared away, in fact it is this minuscule bleeding that forms the black dots often associated with verrucae.

Mosaic warts

Mosaic warts are plaques of myriad small, closely set plantar warts. These warts or verrucae are seldom deeply entrenched but form a matrix like cover over often a quite large area.

Epidermodysplacia Verruciformis (EV)

This disease is by any standard a very rare disease but one that we must be aware of. Its aetiology is multifactorial and displays as lifelong and widespread skin lesions of a persistent nature and is attributed to specific HPV types. The fact that the patient may display normal resistance to other virus, fungal and bacterial infections seems to indicate that their immune system does not respond to these specific HPVs while it may respond to other PVG virus very well.

Although Kremdorf et al identified 15 HPV types in EV lesions there appears to be only one or two found in healthy individuals suffering from EV; of these HPV8 seems to be the leading contender.

When patients presenting with EV are challenged with HPV1, for example, their antibody response may be the same as a person not suffering from EV: that is normal. In EV specific viral infections, however, along with reduced cell mediated immunity, sufferers produce little or no precipitating antibody to the types of HPV present in their lesions. This suggests that immuno incompetence is present which prevents recognition and response to these EV specific HPV types. There is the thought of course that in long term HPV infections, antibodies may gradually reduce to levels at which they can no longer be detected. Latent infection seems to have been proved in one study where 10 out of 100 Asymptomatic EV suffers displayed HPV8 antibodies in serum. This HPV8 strain was specific to EV sufferers and has not been known to cause pathology in normal subjects. This does not however mean that PVG recurrent infections cannot occur in non-EV HPV patients.

Recurrent infection

There is no doubt that many patients do present with what appear to be recurrent HPV infections which simply seem to defy all attempts at a long term cure. Most podiatrists will admit to having battled with many such cases. These patients seem to form the 30% of patients who despite our best intentions and all the chemicals, and other treatment thrown at them, retain infections which will i away permanently (it does seem from studies that the best success we might expect is around 70%). This begs the question: "Why does this occur?" A study conducted by Ferenczy et al may hold the answer. Biopsies of healthy tissue from 5 mm and 10 mm beyond the surgical margins of genital warts of 20 female patients were taken. In 9 cases HPV DNA was detected in samples taken from one or both sites. Six of these patients (66%) had a recurrence of their lesions after treatment compared with only one recurrence in eleven subjects whose biopsies were negative for HPV DNA. Failure therefore to fully encapsulate or remove isolated HPV infections may well explain in some part the recurrence of HPV infections in some if not most of that elusive 30% who refuse to be cured. The fact that the HPV infection can remain latent sometimes for many years has also led to the thought that there may be a trigger mechanism responsible for turning what was a non active disease into an active disease. Much more research needs to be undertaken in this field. Hopefully this will lead to a fuller understanding and better treatment regimes.

Long Standing Plantar Warts (a note of warning)

Plantar Verrucous Carcinoma (PVC)

Studies undertaken seem to demonstrate that in certain longstanding resistant plantar warts, those of 10 years duration or over where treatment both of an aggressive and non-aggressive nature have taken place and particularly those which in the past have been treated with X-ray therapies, may in fact be plantar verrucous carcinoma (PVC). Unsuccessful treatment with X-ray and also it is thought exposure to large amounts of ultraviolet light may in some circumstances turn a resistant wart into a low grade squamus cell carcinoma.

As a PVC cannot be visually differentiated from a plantar wart, it may be the case that a clinician, upon being presented with a long term plantar wart which has seemed to be resistant to many forms of treatment from perhaps many different clinicians over a long period of time, may well feel the need to refer this type of patient for Moh's micrographic chemo-surgery at a hospital dermatology department where it is claimed a success rate of up 98% is possible.

Treatment of Warts (Verrucae)

Before determining the type of treatment to use, several things about the patient have to be taken into account.

a) The age of the patient eg. very old/very young.

b) The general mobility of the patient: can they get to the surgery at the required time?

c) Are they involved in sports that will cause any dressing you may apply to move, thereby causing destruction of healthy tissue?

d) Are they in a position with regard to sports, whereby it would be impossible to keep the dressing dry?

e) What is their pain threshold like? Can they stand the sometimes intense irritation caused by some forms of treatment?

f) What type of verruca is it, large, small, deep, shallow, widespread (as in mosaic)?

g) If it is necessary, can the patient realistically keep the dressing dry for the required length of time (which can be up to seven days)?

h) Is the patient suffering from any medical disability (is he/she a diabetic)?

i) Does the patient have any allergies that may affect treatment? (Allergy to aspirin would negate the use of salicylic acid. Allergy to zinc oxide would determine what types of dressing you decide to use.)

Care should also be used when describing the type of treatment to be administered. The chiropodist and all of his/her staff should be aware that terms that we may have come to use, or that have become common place, may instil at the least unease, at the most outright fear in our patient, eg. the kind chiropodist will BURN IT OUT FOR YOU.

Types of Treatment

Drugs

Bleomycin

Several new methods, whose long-term value and risks are not fully known, are available. One of these, intralesional injection of small amounts of 0.1% solution of Bleomycin in saline, often produces necrosis and cures even stubborn plantar warts. However reports of scleroderma of fingers where warts have been injected with Bleomycin would caution, in spite of its popularity and effectiveness, its use.

Isotretinoin, Etretinate

Extensive warts, even in hitherto untreatable epidermodysplasia verruciformis, have improved or cleared with oral isotretinoin, or etretinate, which must be used by physicians familiar with these drugs and their possible side effects, especially foetal abnormalities if used during pregnancy.

Interferon

Interferon, especially a-interferon intralesionally, or IM, has also cleared intractable lesions of the skin and genitals. Its optimal administration and long term results are under study in several countries.

X-ray Therapy

X-ray therapy has no place in treating warts because of its potential to make them malignant; even in squamous cell carcinomas, which occur in patients with the rare epidermodysplasia verruciformis (EDV). X-ray therapy causes warts to become much more invasive. Ultraviolet exposure is also a potent cocarcinogen in patients with EDV or immunosuppresion for any reason.

Electro-surgery and Fulguration

Both of these methods require the administration of a local anaesthetic under the lesion.

The apparatus usually allows for adjustment of the amount of current used both for excising and cauterizing.

Electro-surgery

On some units the earth pole is allowed to come into contact with the foot or lower leg (usually resting the leg on top of the earth pole). The live end, in the form of a hand piece to which several different probes can be attached, is then used to excise the verruca.

It is usual to use a probe that looks like a round circle of very fine wire attached to the end of a probe. This is gently allowed to come into contact with the skin adjacent to the verruca on its outer extremity, with a slight downward movement drawing the wire down and under the verruca and then up and out of the other side. This with skill, excises the verruca in one go, while at the same time working as a coagulator so that little or no blood loss is experienced.

Very little scar tissue results. The resultant wound should be treated as a burn. The patient experiences little after pain.

Fulguration

Many electro-surgery units also allow for fulguration. Using the same earthing system and probe the unit is switched over to fulguration.

A probe is fitted that looks very like a short piece of wire. This is brought near to the lesion (it does not ever touch the lesion). The current bridges the small gap between probe and lesion, and in so doing creates a spark much like that of an electric welding unit (only minutely so).

As with electro-surgery a local anaesthetic is required.

The resultant wound should be treated as a burn.

Little scar tissue results.

The patient experiences little post-operative pain.

Cryosurgery

Crysosurgery uses nitrous oxide (laughing gas), which is allowed to travel through a gun via plastic tubing, to which can be attached probes of various sizes.

Due to the design of the equipment the probe is allowed to reach about minus 90 deg. C.

When human tissue is frozen, the formation of crystals of water destroys tissue structure and cells die. By introducing an extremely cold probe onto a target site (using KY jelly), a precise area of tissue can be destroyed without damage to surrounding cells. The patient is aware of the treatment, which can prove to be quite painful dependent on the length of time the probe is left in skin contact.

Used gas is exhausted through a tube; this should be exhausted into open air (via a suitable window).

The length of time the probe is left in skin contact will depend on the size of lesion, length of time the lesion has existed, and finally how much discomfort your patient is prepared to put up with. Very often the thawing period is as painful, if not more so than the freezing period.

Liquid nitrogen cryosurgery apparatus

The use of liquid nitrogen through this apparatus allows the practitioner to freeze to much lower temperature – approx. -190 deg. C.

The equipment consists of a cryo-jet flask and trigger head.

Liquid nitrogen can be used to super cool various different sized probes, or can be sprayed direct onto lesions through a selection of nozzles.

Due to the extremely low temperature, and the speed at which a freeze is obtained, the patient appears to suffer slightly less than with conventional freezing techniques.

Against this, however, is the need to keep in stock large amounts of liquid nitrogen. This is normally stored in a large Dewar (specialised container). Because this has to be vented, approx. 0.20 litres per day will be lost due to evaporation. Only clinics with a very large through-put of verruca patients could afford the loss involved in this venting process.

Return period

Where freezing using a probe has taken place a return period of between two to three weeks is usual. In many cases necrotic tissue may by this time have fallen off.

A bursa can sometimes develop underneath the verruca (being filled with serum, or blood and serum). It is better to leave this to disperse naturally as this may well assist in providing the patient with immunity in the future.

In cases where cryosurgery appears to have no effect the operator must think about how they are using the system. For destruction of tissue to occur the area must reach the temperature at which skin tissue dies. While the probe may well reach -90 deg., if the lesion is deep enough it may take some time for the tissue to reach the required temperature due to normal body heat generated by surrounding tissue. If sufficient necrotic tissue has not been removed it may never reach the required temperature. For this reason it may be necessary to remove the upper layers of skin with chemical cautery before resorting to cryosurgery.

Chemical Cautery

Wherever possible caustics which are rapid in action and cause speedy necrosis should be used. This causes complete separation from surrounding tissue and therefore lessens the chance of frequent recurrence.

Some drugs/chemicals, cause suppuration, some maceration, yet others may cause ulceration, causing the verruca to be pushed upwards by the introduction of a bursa of serum under the verruca.

The type of drug/chemical you use will be determined by:

>the return period involved

>the action of the drug/chemical ie ulceration, suppuration etc;

plus all the reasons already stated (age, keeping area dry etc.).

Some of the products that can be used

Dichloroacetic acid	Formaldehyde
Glacial acetic acid	Lactic acid
Monochloroacetic acid	Nitric acid
Parahydroxybenzoic acid	Phenol (carbolic acid)
Podophyllum resin	Potassium hydroxide
Pyrogallic acid	Salicylic acid
Silver nitrate	Trichloroacetic acid
Tri-acid	Proprietary drugs

Use of Drugs in Chemical Cautery

Great care must always be taken when using these materials.

Where these materials are discussed, it is presumed that the operating site has been cleaned thoroughly and is sterile.

Where products that require the site to be masked, that is, products that are designed to stay in place for one week or a prescribed period of time, the writer presumes that this will be done, and will not take up undue space by repeating this each time.

Where these materials are used, it is presumed that as much necrotic tissue as possible has been removed without damage to underlying tissue prior to treatment.

Masking material should be of sufficient thickness to retain the drug/chemical used, and should be applied firmly, taking care that only material that the patient is not allergic to is used.

Where these drugs/chemicals are used, it is presumed that a full case history has been taken that would show up any need to preclude the use of such drugs or dressings as might cause an unwanted reaction in the patient.

Where these drugs/chemicals are used, it is presumed that FULL WRITTEN INSTRUCTIONS outlining what reaction the patient can expect, what to do should any problems occur, along with instructions with regard to keeping the dressing dry where appropriate, have been given to the patient, and that his/her record card is so documented.

Where these drugs/chemicals are used, it is presumed that the practitioner will have taken all precautions (including any not mentioned herein) to ensure the comfort and SAFE treatment of his/her patient.

Dichloroacetic acid

Dichloroacetic acid $CHC_{12}.COOH$ is a colourless liquid with the characteristic vinegary odour of the chloroacetic acids.

Dichloroacetic acid is caustic and keratolytic and is used in the treatment of warts, verrucae and callus.

Dichloroacetic acid is quite mild in use. For verrucae it is often better used with other acids (see Tri-acid).

For the Treatment of Callus

Remove as much as possible of the callus with a scalpel. Paint round the callus with Tinc. Benz. and then mask area. Paint the area to be treated with dichloroacetic acid and allow it to dry.

Cover the callus with suitable dressing.

Return period is around 7 to 10 days.

A cheesy, dirty-looking coagulum will be seen, the edges of which may have started to separate if left up to 14 days. The coagulum may be removed quite easily with a scalpel and in some cases may be partially removed with the dressing, or sometimes simply peeled off. This treatment may be repeated several times dependent on the size and thickness of the callus. This is particularly useful in the treatment of very heavy callus including those associated with hyperhidrosis (excessive sweating).

Formaldehyde

Formaldehyde, H.CHO is a gas prepared by the oxidation of methyl alcohol with atmospheric oxygen using copper as a catalyst.

Some methyl alcohol is left in the product in order to prevent polymerisation.

Formaldehyde solution (liquor Formaldehydi) BP is known in Great Britain and Northern Ireland as FORMALIN and is a saturated solution of the gas in water and contains 37-41% of H.CHO.

'1% solution of formalin' and '1% of formaldehyde' both indicate 1% of this solution.

Formaldehyde solution is a colourless liquid with a pungent odour and a burning taste, miscible in water and alcohol in all proportions. A white deposit may form on storage.

Formalin is astringent, disinfectant and fungicidal. It has the effect of hardening the skin and reducing the apparent secretion of sweat.

The patient may use suspension of a 3-5 % solution daily, painting the lesion area. The patient returns to the surgery for removal of hardened tissue. A smear of petroleum jelly around the site protects the healthy skin.

A 40% solution applied in the surgery is a better way to use this product. Painted onto the site by the practitioner. Return period 7 days.

Particularly useful where ulceration and/or suppuration are contraindicated.

For use in sterilising shoes: place the shoes in a plastic bag and inside the bag place a small jar of formalin. Close the bag and leave for 24 hours if possible, if not overnight.

For use in sterilising boots: place a swab of cotton wool soaked in formalin in the boot and enclose in clingfilm for 24 hours if possible, if not overnight.

Glacial acetic acid

Glacial acetic acid contains no less than 99% of CH$_3$.COOH. Acetic acid is converted to sodium acetate, distilled with sulphuric acid and purified by freezing. It is a clear, colourless liquid with a distinctive vinegary odour.

Below 14° C it crystallises to form colourless crystals. On very cold days it may be necessary to warm the bottle before use.

Water should never be added to dissolve the crystals.

Glacial acetic acid is a weak acid which may be rubefacient, vesicant or caustic dependent on the length of time it is in contact with the skin. It may be used as a paint in the treatment of hard or vascular corns, or of verruca pedis.

A method of treatment in the case of verrucae is, first, to saturate the growth with the product, which should be rubbed well in, and then to rub the growth with a stick of silver nitrate BP which has been moistened with water. Two or three further applications of glacial acetic acid are made alternately with silver nitrate, to complete a single treatment.

Minimum return period 4 days.

Glacial acetic acid may also be used as a neutralising agent following treatment of verrucae with potassium hydroxide (see potassium hydroxide).

Lactic acid

Lactic acid is a colourless syrupy liquid with a sour taste, containing not less than the equivalent of 87.5% w/w of $CH_3CHOH.COOH$. It is miscible in water and alcohol and mixes well with glycerine.

Lactic Acid is keratolytic on thickened epidermis and an ointment containing 20-30% may be used in the treatment of corns and warts/verrucae.

Lactic Acid is not widely used by itself in chiropody.

Its use with other acids is quite popular however due to its mild action e.g. below.

Lactic acid 25% and salicylic acid 25%

This treatment is quite mild in action, and as such is suitable for the very young/old.

Mask and apply as with other ointments.

Keep dry until return.

Return period is 7 days.

Monochloroacetic acid

Monochloroacetic acid $CH_2C_1.COOH$ occurs as deliquescent crystals, which are readily soluble in water, alcohol and ether.

It is made by passing chlorine into acetic acid in the presence of sunlight or iodine.

It acts by hydrolysing protein, and is very penetrating. Action can be checked by the application of compresses of saturated solution of sodium bicarbonate or neutralised before absorption by irrigation with a solution of potassium hydroxide.

Great care must be taken in the use, and handling, of this product.

Monochloroacetic acid is very caustic and may cause burns to the hands if not used correctly.

Method 1: using the product by itself

A saturated solution of the product is applied to the growth with a cotton bud.

The patient keeps the area dry and returns in 2/3 days when necrotic tissue is removed. The product is then re-applied etc.

Method 2

A second way of using the product is to rub a crystal of monochloroacetic acid into the growth for a timed period. The dosage will vary according to the duration of the application: 30-60 seconds is suggested as an experimental starting point.

Return period 7 days.

In both the above treatments the foot must be kept dry between visits.

Breakdown can be expected and there may be some pain. The methods are contraindicated where breakdown is to be avoided. Monochloroacetic acid can be used with other products (see salicylic acid).

Nitric acid

Nitric acid is a colourless liquid that fumes on exposure to air. It contains 70% of HNO_3. It should be stored in glass-stoppered containers. It should be stored well away from any metallic objects.

Nitric acid is caustic with a powerful oxidising action. It does not readily dissolve the precipitated proteins, thus its action is more circumscribed than either sulphuric or hydrochloric acid. It stains the skin yellow but does not char the tissue. It is used for the treatment of warts and occasionally vascular corns and hypergranulation tissue as well as verrucae. It is a powerful caustic on account of its oxidising power and because it coagulates proteins. It is to be preferred to sulphuric and hydrochloric acids in the treatment of verrucae, but should be used with great care. Daily treatments should be given. The coagulated tissue should be removed weekly.

Method 1

After the removal of the superficial layers of verrucae, nitric acid is applied using a glass rod or an orange stick with a little cotton wool wound around it. The acid is left on the verrucae for about 5 minutes and its action is then stopped by means of a 10% solution of phenol. The skin will be stained a bright yellow owing to the formation of trinitrophenol. The phenol will also serve to reduce the pain caused by the action of the nitric acid.

Method 2

After operating, the growth is first saturated with 5% phenol for 5 minutes. Nitric acid is then applied to the verrucae and left on for 15-25 seconds. The growth is again saturated with 5% phenol. This method obviates much of the pain that might otherwise be felt due to the nitric acid.

In both these methods each application is complete in itself. Both methods are useful where rapid results are called for.

Please note: because nitric acid fumes when exposed to air, it has the appearance of a very strong acid and this may frighten nervous patients or children.

Parahydroxybenzoic acid

Parahydroxybenzoic acid is a close chemical relative of salicylic acid, differing from it only in the relative positions of the -OH and -COOH radicals in the benzene ring.

Parahydroxybenzoic acid produces a drier coagulum than salicylic and appears to cause less maceration of surrounding tissues.

It may be used instead of salicylic acid in the treatment of corns and warts/verrucae, in the same strengths as salicylic acid.

It does not appear to cause a breakdown of tissue in the same way that salicylic acid may do when used on warts/verrucae.

It may also be used with monochloroacetic acid in much the same way as salicylic acid.

Phenol (carbolic acid)

Carbolic acid is hydroxybenzene and occurs as colourless needle-shaped, deliquescent crystals which become pinkish on keeping, and which contain not less than 98% of C_6H_5OH. Soluble in water, alcohol, ether, benzol, chloroform, carbon bisulphide, glycerine, and fixed in volatile oils, mineral oils, soft paraffin, and alkaline solutions.

Phenol should be stored in a cool dark place in a brown glass sealed container.

Phenol is analgesic and caustic and must always be used with care owing to its caustic properties and due to the fact that it causes constriction of the smaller blood vessels when applied as a wet dressing and tends, on account of its analgesic properties, to cause painless gangrene.

Phenol paralyses the sensory nerve endings in the skin and is used as an analgesic in cases of pruritis and also, on occasions, to alleviate the pain when operating on a hard corn and/or verrucae.

Phenol is more usually used with other preparations in the treatment of verrucae (see salicylic acid).

When phenol has turned a pink colour it is old and should be discarded. Owing to its oxidising action, it has a very superficial action on the skin when applied in small doses.

Pyrogallic acid

Colourless crystals, which become brown coloured on exposure to light and air. Should be stored in amber coloured bottles. Readily soluble in water.

Pyrogallic acid produces a dark brown eschar. It appears to have analgesic properties.

A powerful antiseptic due to its affinity for oxygen.

It is used as a parasiticide, and is used in ointment form to treat ringworm, psoriasis, chronic eczema, etc.

It has a tendency to stain the hair and skin black. The stain may be removed by ammonium persulphate.

Great care should be taken in using this product as it does have a cumulative effect and can cause poisoning by absorption.

The formulae for pyrogallol are very similar to that of phenol. No doubt because of this does seem to enjoy analgesic properties and is particularly useful in treating neuro-vascular verrucae, and in weaker strengths also for treatment of painful corns.

For treatment to verrucae, strengths of up to 50% in white soft paraffin wax.

For use with painful corns, around 20% in ointment base.

Up to 70% strength can be used under controlled conditions, but only as a one off treatment (due to cumulative effect).

Contraindication: in cases where the skin is very moist or very dry, with elderly or diabetic patients, and where circulation or underlying tissue is inadequate.

Return period 7 days. Keep dry.

Please note: at the best it is generally thought that this product should be used NOT MORE THAN TWICE. At the worst it is thought by some to be a carcinogen.

Podophyllum resin

Podophyllum resin is a mixture of resins from the dried rhizome and roots of Podophyllum pelatum or Hexandrum.

It is a light brown powder. Since it is very irritant to the eyes care should be taken when the powder is being handled.

As paint, it is made up from 15% podophyllum, and made up to 100% with compound benzoin.

Podophyllum ointment

As in Vericap and Posafilin: both contain 20% Podophyllum and 25% salicylic acid.

They tend to be self-administered by the patient. They can have some uses in the treatment of mosaic warts/verrucae.

Potassium hydroxide (alkaline)

Potassium hydroxide occurs as a white deliquescent cake or pellet and contains not less than 85% KOH.

It is strongly alkaline and corrosive, destroying organic tissues rapidly. It is very soluble in water, alcohol and glycerine. It absorbs carbon dioxide from the air and should be stored in well-closed containers.

Great care should be taken using this alkaline product.

Never touch the pellets with the fingers, as alkaline burns will occur.

Pare away the superficial layers of tissue.

Immerse the foot in a bath of warm water for 5 minutes.

Dry the foot and then rub a pellet of KOH gently into the growth (the pellet should be held in forceps, preferably plastic).

The foot is now immersed in water again for about 2 minutes.

Following this immersion a jelly-like material will be found to have formed over the growth. This should be scraped away.

The foot may be treated several times dependent on size of growth etc.

The growth is treated with glacial acetic acid to neutralise the alkaline.

There is no return period as each treatment is complete in itself.

Indications: when conventional treatments have failed to work, or on obstinate growths. Where rapid results are required.

Contraindications: in cases of poor circulation, or when the patient does not enjoy good general health, or on very shallow growths where there is little underlying tissue.

Salicylic acid

Salicylic Acid is ortho-hydroxybenzoic acid, containing not less than 99.5% of $C_6H_4.OH.COOH$. It occurs as colourless, needle shaped crystals, or as light, feathery powder. Odourless, with a sweet, acrid taste. Soluble in water, ether, or alcohol.

Action and uses: antiseptic and caustic, slightly irritant and keratolytic. Less necrotic than phenol, but when used in strong solution, or ointment form, must be applied with care.

Can be used as a dusting powder in the treatment of dermatitis, bromidrosis, hyperhidrosis, maceration etc. 3% in powder.

Usually used in an ointment base in strengths from 20% to 70% in the treatment of hard corns and verrucae.

Salicylic acid can also be used in conjunction with other drugs/chemicals.

On moderately severe verrucae, mask; apply 70% salicylic acid paste. Keep dry for 7 days. Upon return, remove necrotic tissue and re-treat: this treatment may be the same or a lesser strength, or silver nitrate 90%.

On severe or intractable cases, soak a cotton bud with liquefied phenol 80%; rub this into the verruca for 4 minutes.

Wash off with isopropyl alcohol.

Mask with suitable thickness dressing. Fill the aperture in the dressing with 70% salicylic acid paste.

Press one sugar sized crystal of monochloroacetic acid into the paste.

Return period is 7 days. Keep dry.

Alternatively, you may mix several crystals of monochloroacetic acid into a small amount of salicylic acid paste, reserving this for just such an occasion.

Follow procedure above to masking stage.

Apply a little of the pre-mixed paste first, followed by 70% paste.

Return period is 7 days. Keep Dry.

Please note that monochloroacetic acid crystals should be handled with extreme care: they are very caustic.

Protect hands from contact with product.

Follow precautions on the container.

In the above-mentioned methods the phenol appears to work as a type of wetting agent, penetrating the tissue. The monochloroacetic acid responds to the heat of the foot, dissolving, and appears to penetrate the tissue as did the phenol. This continues for approx. two days. The analgesic property of the phenol does appear to help with pain control.

In the meantime the salicylic acid, slower in reaction, begins to work, continuing to destroy tissue, as has the monochloroacetic acid and phenol, causing maceration.

Ulceration and breakdown can occur (the treatment is contraindicated where breakdown would be harmful to the patient). Should this occur, soak the foot in salt water.

Leave for at least 24 hours if possible before attempting to clear the area.

As with any acid preparation the antidote is a mild alkali such as potassium hydroxide solution 5%. Painted onto the area this will help to neutralise the acids you have applied.

Silver nitrate

Silver nitrate occurs as colourless tabular crystals with a bitter metallic taste, containing not less than 99.8% of $AgNO_3$.

It should be stored away from the light, in glass stoppered bottles.

It is soluble 2 parts in 1 part water, and 1 in 27 of 95% alcohol.

Antidote: the immediate application of a compress of a 10% aqueous solution of sodium chloride or footbath of a strong saline solution will relieve pain due to silver nitrate.

Patients with fair skin tend to react severely as do patients with very dry skin: care should be taken with this type of patient.

Of all the products used silver nitrate is perhaps the fastest to induce pain.

The pain experienced with silver nitrate can be extreme; however, it is usually short lived, lasting no longer than 24 hours.

Although the return period is usually 7 days, the foot may be immersed in water after 24 hours as effectively the silver nitrate has stopped working by this time.

A dark, black-looking eschar is apparent after treatment and it is advised that you inform your patient that this will be the case and need not cause undue concern.

Silver nitrate can be used in its liquid form for other treatments in chiropody; however, it is usually used in two forms for verrucae.

> *Toughened silver nitrate* is formed by fusing 95% silver nitrate with 5% potassium nitrate, usually supplied in a special holder.

> *Silver nitrate mitigated* is formed using 33% silver nitrate and potassium nitrate, again supplied in a special holder.

When applied to the skin, it is said that silver nitrate combines with the skin proteins to form a thick layer of silver albumate, which at first turns white, but gradually changes to brown and then to black, under the influence of light. Because it forms an insoluble barrier by combining with the tissue chlorides, silver nitrate does not penetrate deeply.

It would seem that the action of silver nitrate on the skin takes place very rapidly. Even if it is neutralised with sodium chloride immediately after application, a black coagulum will be formed.

Toughened silver nitrate is the product mostly used with regard to verrucae. Although literature says it should be moistened before use, it is better to moisten the lesion and then rub the silver nitrate into the lesion.

Do not use spirits to moisten the lesion as this lessens the effectiveness of this product.

Silver nitrate can be used with other drugs/chemicals (see glacial acetic acid).

Silver nitrate is often used as the final part of the treatment of verrucae because of its ability to stain skin tissue, and show up any verrucae that may still be present, and also because silver nitrate does not penetrate deeply and so may just finish off any last lingering bits that you may not be quite sure about.

Trichloroacetic acid

Trichloroacetic acid occurs as very deliquescent crystals containing not less than 98% of $CCl_3.COOH$.

It should be stored in moisture excluding containers. The crystals are readily soluble in water.

Trichloroacetic acid is caustic, keratolytic and astringent and is used either by itself or with other chemicals in the treatment of verrucae.

Although it is considered chemically stronger than monochloroacetic, it is generally considered that its action is less drastic and more superficial than that of the latter.

This may well be the case if painting onto a lesion; however, use of the crystals as in monochloroacetic acid would make it STRONGER IN USE.

Trichloroacetic acid may be used in the same way as monochloroacetic acid, that is a saturated solution may be painted onto the growth with a cotton bud. Return period not less than 4 days.

A crystal of the product may be rubbed into the growth for a timed period (try 30 seconds as a starting point). This product is much stronger than using a saturated solution. Return period 4-14 days.

After removing the superficial layers, the growth is first soaked with a solution of trichloroacetic acid, and then treated with silver nitrate (toughened). This is repeated until there are several layers of trichloroacetic and silver nitrate.

Unlike the above methods where the foot must be kept dry until the return period, this method allows for the foot to get wet after 24 hours.

Tri-acid

Tri-acid consists of

> three parts monochloroacetic acid
> two parts dichloroacetic acid
> one part trichloroacetic acid

Soak the growth with the concentrate using a cotton bud.

Cover and keep dry.

Return period is 7 days, when a cheesy type of coagulum will have formed.

With care tri-acid can be used with and alongside other products as experience dictates.

Proprietary drugs

The following are usually supplied via the patient's G.P. or can be purchased over the counter and are usually self-administered.

There are many more products on the market than these mentioned. The following drugs are mentioned to give a rough idea of how this type of drug is made up.

Compound V	Whitehall Labs.	Sal.A.Ph.Eur. 17% w/w Acetone BP Pyroxilin BP IMS 99% BP Castor Oil Ph.Eur.
Bazuka-gel (original)	Diomed Developments	Sal.Acid BP 12% w/w Lactic A.BP 4% w/w Camphor BP Pyroxylin BP Ethanol BP Ethyl Acetate
Bazuka-gel (extra strength)	Diomed Developments	Sal.A. 26% w/w Camphor BP Povidone BP Pyroxylin BP Ethanol BP Acetone
Duofilm	Stiefel Labs.	Sal.A.BP 16.7% w/w Lactic A.BP 16.7% Flexible Collodion 66.6% w/w
Glutarol	Dermal Labs.	Paint containing Glutaraldehyde 10% w/w
Posalfilin Ointment	Norgine Ltd	Podophyllum resin BP 20% Sal.A.BP 25%
Salactal Gel	Dermal Labs.	Sal.A.BP 12.0% w/w Lactic A BP 4.0% w/w
Salactol	Dermal Labs.	Sal.A.BP 16.7% w/w Lactic A. 16.7% w/w Flexible Collodion 66.6% w/w
Verucasep Gel	Galen Ltd	Activated Glutaraldehyde 10% w/w

Glossary of Common Terms

Antibody

A body or substance evoked by an antigen, and characterised by reacting specifically with the antigen in some demonstrable way.

Antigen

Allergen, immunogen: any substance that, as a result of coming into contact with appropriate tissues, induces a state of sensitivity and/or resistance to infection or toxic substances after a latent period of 8 to 14 days and which reacts with tissues and/or antibody of the sensitised subject in vivo or in vitro.

CMI

Cell Mediated Immunity

CS

Glucocorticoids

Cytotoxic cells

Detrimental or destructive to cells; pertaining to the effect of noncytophilic antibody on specific antigen, frequently, but not always, mediating the action of complement.

Dendritic cells

Dendritic ('tree-shaped' or 'branching') process; neurodendrite; neurodendron; one of the two types of branching protoplasmic processes of the nerve cell (the other being the axon).

Dermis corium

Cutis vera; enderon; a layer of skin composed of a superficial thin layer that interdigitates with the epidermis, the stratum papillare, and the stratum reticulare; it contains blood and lymphatic vessels, nerves and nerve endings, glands, and except for glabrous skin, hair follicles.

DNA

Deoxyribonucleic acid; the type of nucleic acid containing deoxyribose as the sugar component and found principally in the nuclei (chromantin, chromasomes) of animal and vegetable cells usually loosely bound to protein. Considered to be the auto-reproducing component of chromosomes and many viruses and the repository of hereditary characteristics, in other words the building blocks of life.

Epidermis

The outer epithelial portion of the skin. The palms and soles have the following strata:

a) Stratum corneum (horny layer)
b) Stratum lucidum (clear layer) (in other parts of the body stratum lucidum may not be present)
c) Stratum granulosum (granular layer)
d) Stratum basale (basal layer)

EV

Epidermodysplacia Verruciformis

HPV

Human Papilloma Virus

HPV 1

Plantar warts

HPV 2

Mosaic plantar warts

HPV 4

Palmo/plantar warts (punctate warts)

HPV 8

Epidermodysplacia verruciformis

HPV 16

70% of genital warts

Iatrogenic

Denoting an unfavourable response to medical or surgical treatment induced by the treatment itself.

Interferon

A glycoprotein. Effects include inhibition of cellular growth, alterations in the state of cellular differentiation, effects on cell cycle, interference with oncogen expression, alterations in cell surface antigen expression, effects on antibody production, and regulation of cytotoxic effecter cells.

Interleukin

One of several proteins important for lymphocyte proliferation.

Interleukin-1 (IL1)

Produced by macrophages and induces the production of interleukin–2 by T cells that have been stimulated by antigen or mitogen.

Interleukin-2 (IL2)

Produced by T cells, stimulates the proliferation of T cells bearing specific receptors for IL-2; these receptors are expressed in response to antigen stimulation. IL-2 also seems to induce the production of interferon and is used as an anti-cancer drug in the treatment of a wide variety of solid malignant tumours.

Lymphocytes

White blood cell formed in lymphatic tissue throughout the body.

Lymphocyte B cells

An immunologically important lymphocyte that is not thymus-dependent, is of short life, and is responsible for the production of immunoglobulins. It is the precursor of the plasma cell and does not play a role in cell-mediated immunity.

Macrophage

Any mononuclear, actively phagocytic cell arising from monocytic stem cells in bone marrow; these cells are widely distributed in the body and vary in morphology and motility, though most are large, long lived cells with nearly round nucleus. Phagocytic activity is typically mediated by serum recognition factors, including certain immunoglobulins and components of the complement system but can also be non-specific for some inert materials and bacteria. They are also involved in both the production of antibodies and cell mediated immune responses. They participate in presenting antigens to lymphocytes, and secrete a variety of immunoregulatory molecules.

NK Cells

Langerhans Cells (bone marrow derived) and assume a suprabasilar location within the epidermis. They form a horizontally disposed network of dendritic cells.

Phagocyte

Any cell capable of ingesting particular matter. The term usually refers to two types: polymorphonuclear leukocytes and mononuclear phagocytes (macrophages and monocytes).

PVC

Plantar Verrucous Carcinoma

PVG

Papilloma Virus Group

T cell

A thymocyte-derived lymphocyte of immunological importance that is long lived (months or years) and is responsible for cell mediated immunity.

VP

Verruca Plantaris

VV

Verruca Vulgaris

Photographic Plates

Figures 1-5

We need first to determine if what is present really is a verruca. In this case, treated by a local GP, silver nitrate was used to treat what he perceived to be verrucae. Great damage was done to the patient who eventually attended a chiropodist because she could no longer stand the pain of her GP's treatment. The 'verruca' turned out to be several seed corns. The patient therefore underwent treatment that was both painful and costly – all because of original misdiagnosis.

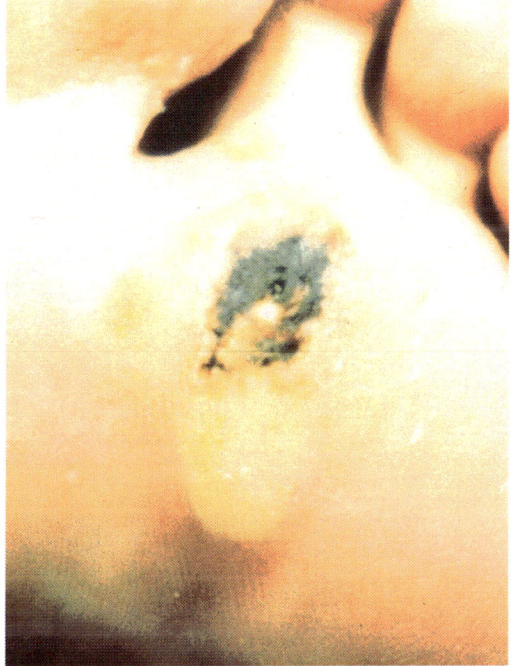

Figure 1

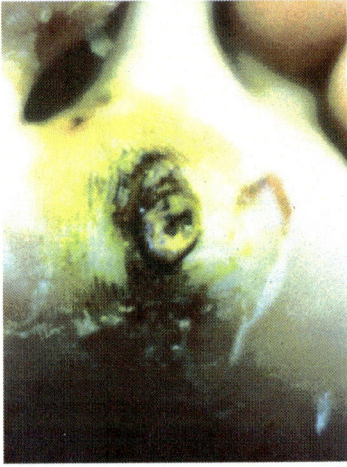

Figure 2

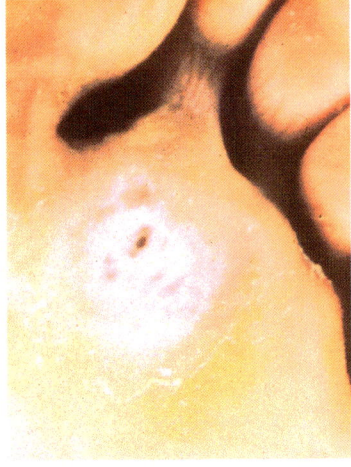

Figure 3

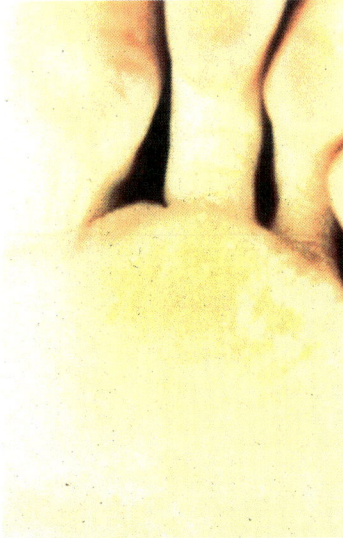

Figure 4

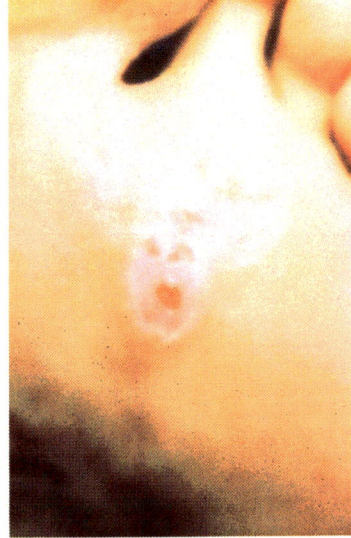

Figure 5

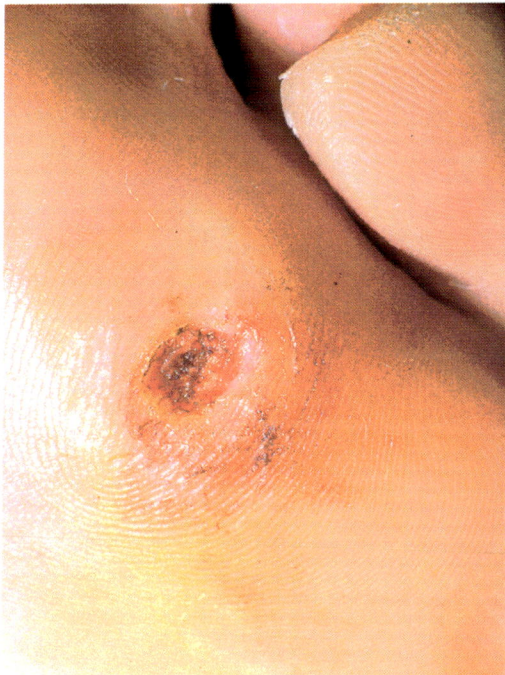

Figure 6

An illustration of what can be achieved with electro-surgery. The verruca was removed seven days before this photograph was taken. An anaesthetic was administered below the verruca which was then removed as completely as possible. The area will feel much as a burn would and will heal with very little scar tissue.

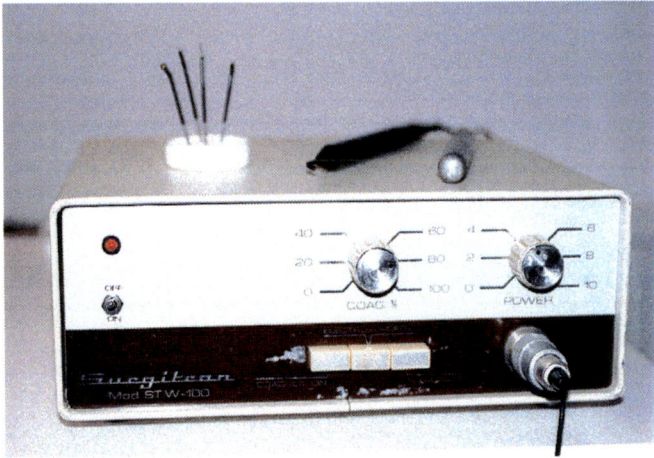

Figure 7

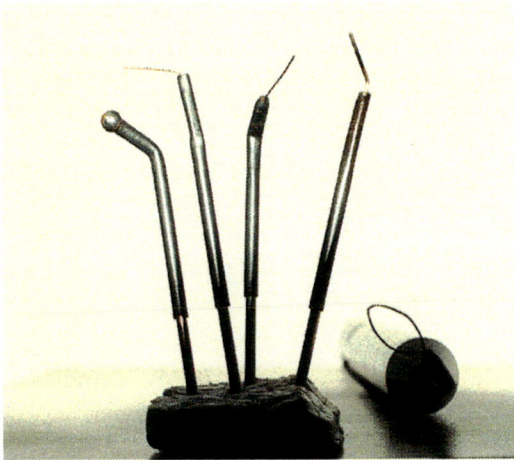

Figure 8

Figures 7 & 8. A typical electro surgery unit. This particular unit can be used to cut using the thinner probes or the circular probe (attached to the handle) as described in the main body of text. The unit can also be used for fulguration using the thicker probes and for coagulation using the ball-like probe.

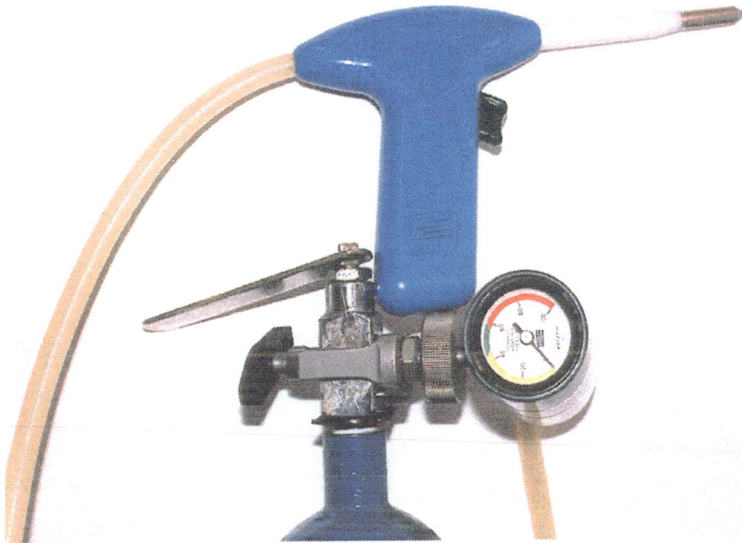

Figure 9. A typical cryosurgery unit utilising a cylinder of nitrous oxide.

Figure 10. The probe can be removed and different size probes fitted. The exhaust tube must be vented outside the room or operating area.

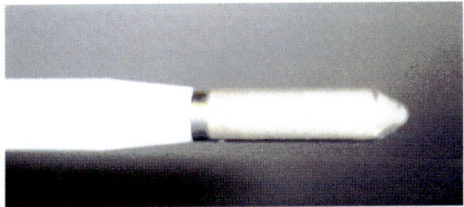

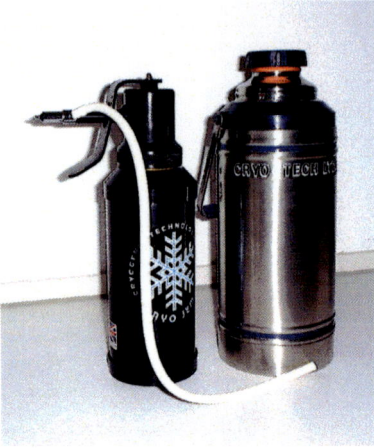

Figure 11 (above). A liquid nitrogen cryo-unit along with a small flask suitable only for moving liquid nitrogen between surgeries.

Figure 12 (right). A large Dewar for holding liquid nitrogen. Liquid nitrogen evaporates, and so quite a substantial amount of the product purchased would be wasted due to evaporation.

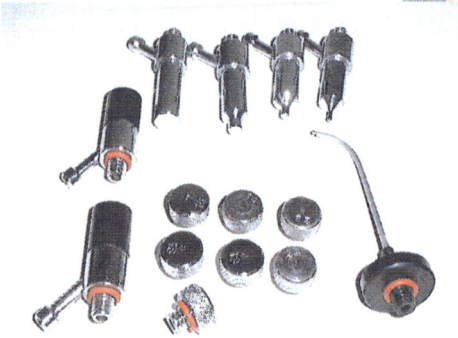

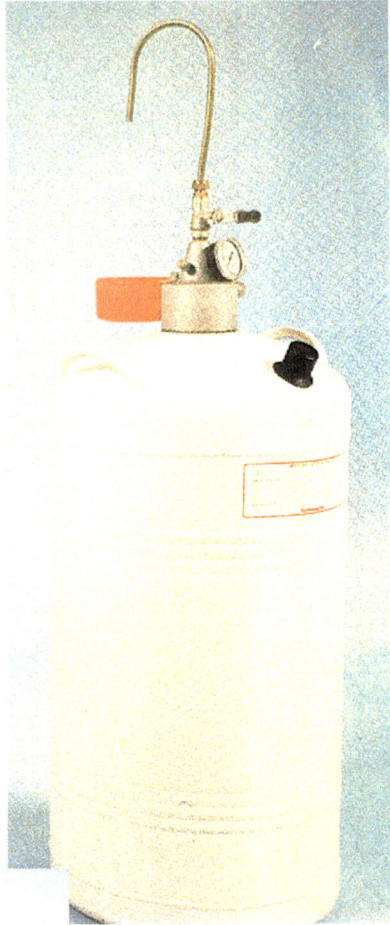

Figure 13 (left). Nozzles (liquid nitrogen can be sprayed with these) for the liquid nitrogen cryo-unti; also probes of different sizes.

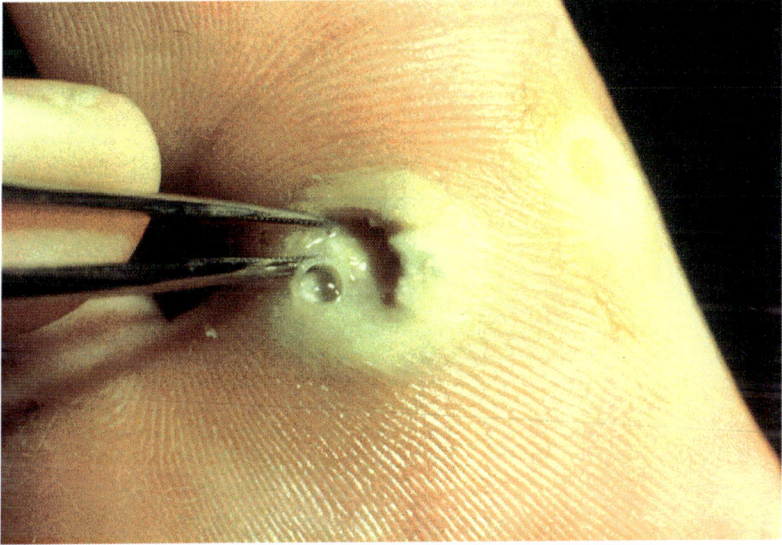

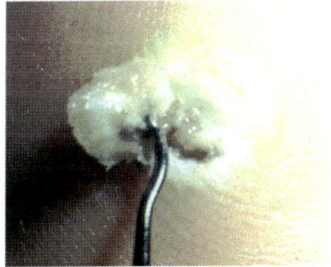

Figure 14 (A and B). Although used in this case to treat a sinus, this is a good example of how important it is to mask really well. The area was first painted with phenol and allowed to soak for two minutes. It was then washed off with alcohol.

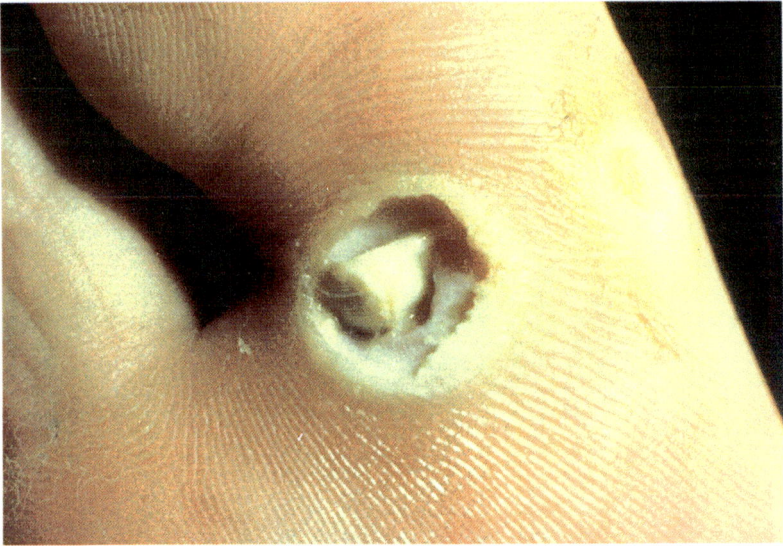

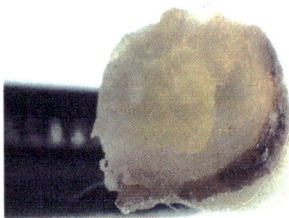

Figure 15 (A and B). The area was then thoroughly masked and 70% sal. and monochloroacetic acid was applied (three crystals). It was then kept dry for 7 days. Because the sinus is more fibrous than normal skin, the skin adjacent to the sinus was attacked, more so than the sinus (see left).

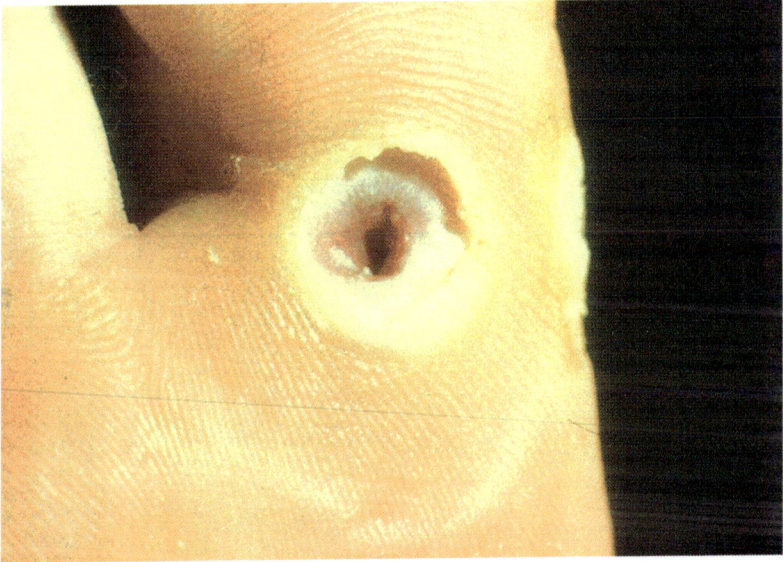

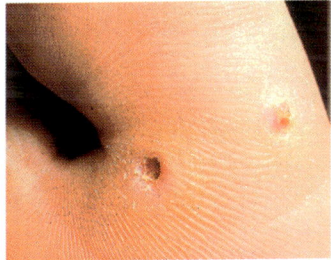

Figure 16 (A and B). After 7 days the necrotic tissue was removed (by this time maceration had taken place). Fluid filled the area separating the sinus from the adjacent tissue, allowing the sinus to be removed. As can be seen, due to an old injury the sinus had to be removed in two pieces, from two different sites.

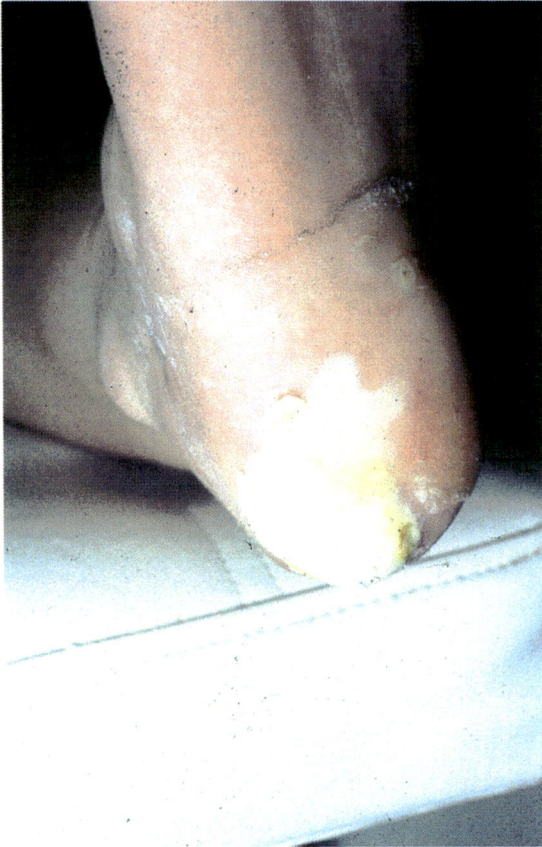

Figure 17. These verrucae presented very much like mosaic verrucae. They were in fact all quite separate and very deep verrucae. Figures 17 - 22 show weekly treatment with salicylic acid at 70% along with a few crystals of monochloroacetic acid.

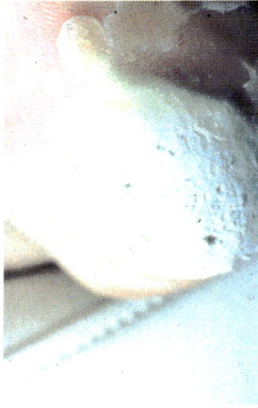

Figure 18

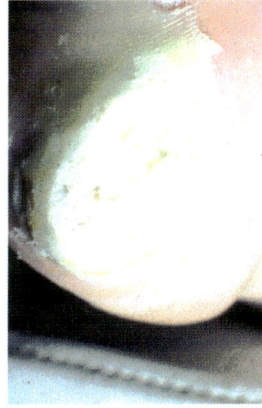

Figure 19

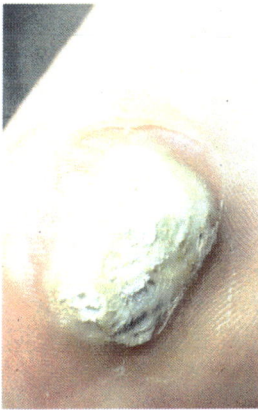

Figure 20

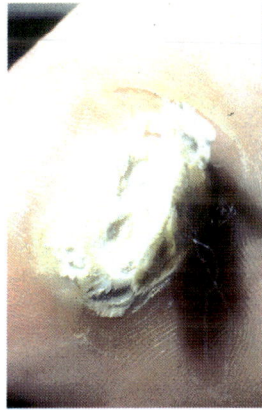

Figure 21

Figures 18 – 21. The gradual reduction of area from the outside edges inwards can be clearly seen with the outer verrucae being the first to go.

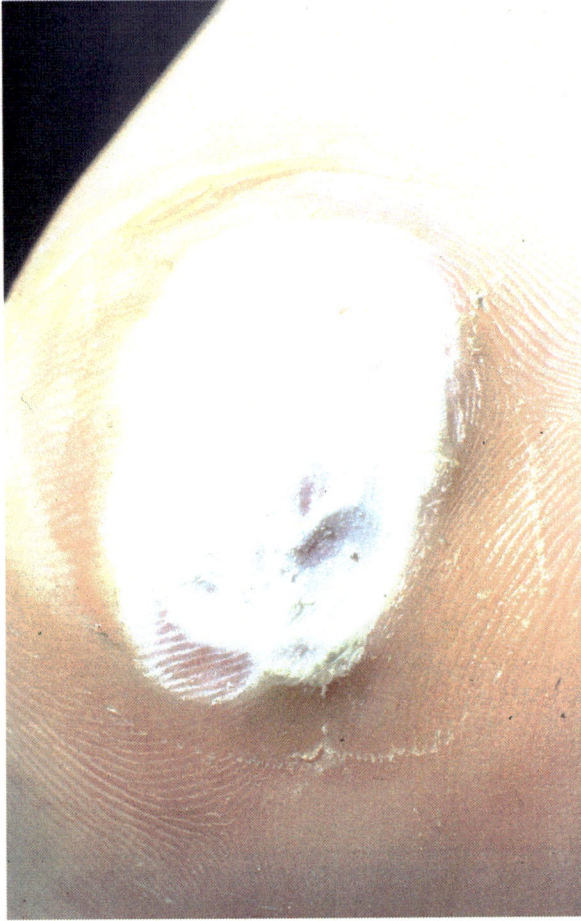

Figure 22. From the above sequence of six figures it can also be seen that a thick pad was used for masking purposes, allowing the plantar skin to be extruded into the pad and thus the medicament applied: this allows the drugs used to penetrate from the top down, and to a certain extent inwards from the sides. A gradual increase of healthy footprint can be observed.

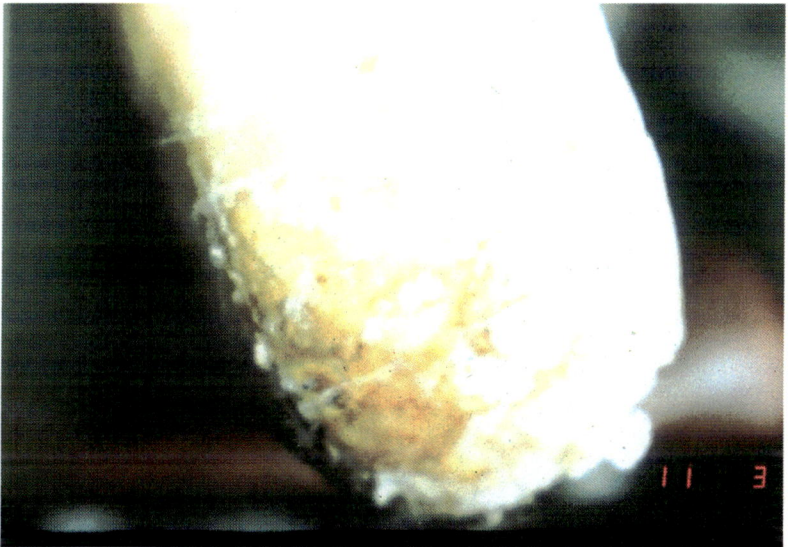

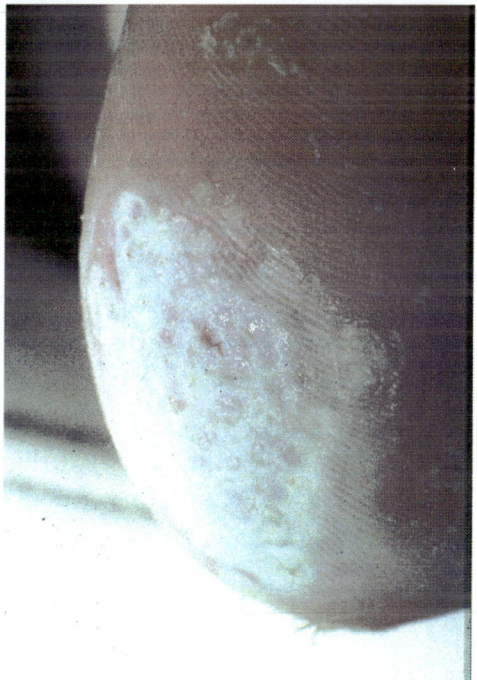

Figure 23 (above). These mosaic verrucae were treated with 70% salicylic acid with a return period of one week.

Figure 24 (right). After one week they were each spotted with a saturated solution of monochloroacetic acid with a return period of two days. The resultant dried eschar was removed before re-applying monochloroacetic acid until the problem had resolved (about four weeks all told).

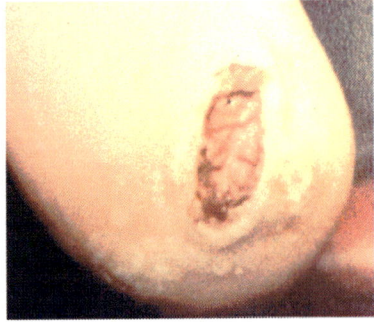

Figure 25. It is said by some that verrucae are very superficial and that they do not go very deep. The picture to the right shows that this is not the case. This verruca has penetrated through both the epidermis and the dermis. The fatty pockets under the skin can be seen quite clearly.

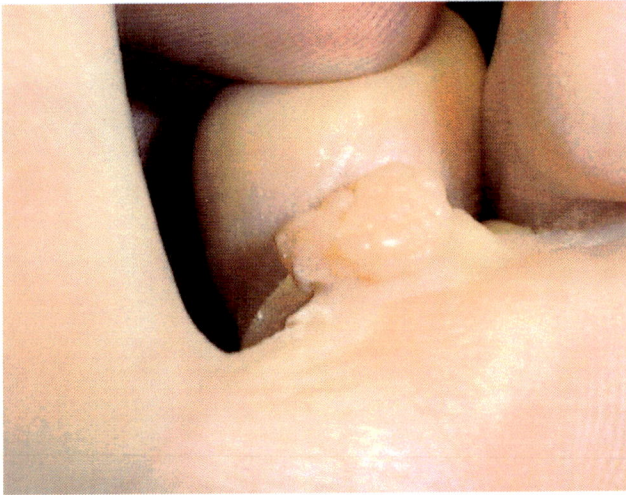

Figure 26. This photograph rather lends a lie to the statement that 'the elderly rarely suffer from HPVG'. This pendunculated wart (resembling a cauliflower) is seen on the head of the second metatarso-phalangeal joint of a 68 year old woman.